My Battles With
And
Victory Over
Severe Sickness

Clairgar Cooke-Robertson

Cover designed by Jenness Reid

All scripture quotations are taken from The Holy Bible,
King James Version (KJV) – public domain.

Clairgar Cooke-Robertson
Email: ClairgarCook@gmail.com or,
tyronetrroberts10@gmail.com.

Printed in the United States of America

First Printing: October 2018

ISBN-13 978-1-7241937-5-9

Dedication

I dedicate this book to all those who are going through severe sicknesses. May they find strength in Jesus Christ of Nazareth, as they read this book.

Contents

Acknowledgement

First, I give thanks to God for helping me when I was going through my severe sickness.

Thanks to all the doctors, nurses, nurse aides, and family members who inspired me and provided care during my sickness. Without God and their help, I could not survive to tell my story. Special thanks to my kidney donor who, although anonymous, was kind enough to give me one of his kidneys. My God bless his heart.

Preface

It is never easy to hear that you have been diagnosed with a severe sickness. It can have consequences beyond your imagination. Your lifestyle can change – eating habits, what you do daily, your work performance and even being able to continue working.

The impact of being diagnosed with a severe sickness also extends to your family. Before the diagnosis, you might have been the main caregiver. However, this can change quickly and instead you must depend on family to provide care – morally, financially or physically, so that you can endure and overcome the sickness. There is strength in unity; so, if family members join you in the fight to overcome the sickness, your chances of surviving are much greater.

If diagnosed with a severe sickness, how you handle it determines the outcome. In my case, even though I followed up with the doctors and other caregivers, I looked to my Eternal Father in Heaven to direct my medical help, through them.

I know that my Eternal Father created me, so He knows how to fix all that is going wrong in my body. The knowledge that I belong to my Heavenly Father, the many prayers that went up to Him for me by others, myself, and my beloved family have helped in my health's successful recovery.

I was inspired by my Heavenly Father to write this book to help others and their family who might be facing the challenges of severe sicknesses. If you are in this situation, I encourage you to have faith and to reach out to your Eternal Father for help. God answers all sincere prayers.

Chapter 1

Onset Of The Sickness

I originated from Jamaica, West Indies. I have six children. Three boys (Lee, Everton, and Tyrone) and Three girls (Sophia, Diane, and Nashera). After my husband, passed away in 1996, I had to take care of the children on my own. I became mother and father to them. I have a beautiful family in which I was the main caregiver.

I had the opportunity to work in the Bahamas; so, I lived there for 15 years before migrating to the United States in 1983. In the United States, I first worked as a Home Health Aide then later at United Cerebral Palsy (UCP) facility. There I administered medications and general care to the patients.

In 2001, while working at Wayne Nursing Home in the Bronx, I experienced early sign of what ended up been a debilitating sickness. I distinctly remembered that I bought a cup of coffee and was about to sip it when a coworker requested that I help her to move a patient. I put the coffee down and assisted her.

After caring for the patient, I went and got my cup of coffee. I took a sip. It tasted odd, so, I threw it away. Later that day, my feet started swelling. I thought it happened because I was working long hours standing on them.

While having lunch with my coworker that day, I mentioned to her that my feet was swelling. She said to me, "Clair, when you go home, elevate your feet in the air and watch to see if the swelling goes down." At home, I soaked my feet in Epsom salt dissolved in warm water and then rub them with alcohol. Next, I used two pillows to elevate my feet. After this treatment, the swelling went down a little.

I returned to work, on the 3:00 p.m. to 11:00 p.m. shift. However, the swelling would not go down, so I decided to see a doctor. I looked up a doctor who was participating in my health insurance and went to consult him. He thought the swelling might be due to arthritis. He did not give me any medication to treat the condition. So, the swelling problem persisted. I began to get very worried. My children encouraged me to seek a second opinion.

I went to Dr. Van Hook and she decided to investigate more. She sent me for blood and urine tests. About a week later, she called and told me to come and see her for the tests results. I got very nervous because I was apprehensive of the results. I had diarrhea due to nervous reaction. All kinds of thoughts were crossing my mind, "Could it be aids, cancer, or something else. What is going on in my body?" While still on the toilet, I received a phone call from my daughter, Sophia.

I told Sophia that I had to go and see the doctor for the tests results. She asked for the doctor's number and I gave it to her. She called the doctor and then called me back. She told me to go to the car, pray, and then drive to the doctor's office.

I went to the car and prayed. I asked God to be my leader and declared that I was the follower. I asked for strength to face the doctor and hear about what was going on with my health. I told God He was in control with what was going on with my health.

Chapter 2

The Diagnosis

I reached the doctor's office late. However, I was much less nervous about what I could be hearing because I had prayed and called on my Heavenly Father to take control of my health situation.

When I went in to see Dr. Van Hook she explained the blood test and urine test results. She stated that the results showed I had "lupus" and it was interfering with my kidney. She recommended that I see Dr. Robert Lynn who was a kidney specialist. I immediately became worried, stressed and depressed. I did not know what to do. I had no idea what she was talking about. No one in the family had lupus, so it was strange to me. I had to excuse myself and go to the bathroom.

I called my daughter, Sophia, and told her what Dr. Van Hook said. My daughter was astonished and began crying. She told me to ask the doctor to explain to me what lupus really was.

After composing myself a little, I returned to talk to Dr. Van Hook. I asked her to fully explain to me what lupus is. She said, "It is a disease that attacks the kidneys where the red blood cells destroy the white blood cells." She further told me not to worry about the test. She stated that I should get on the dialysis machine and clean my blood and that it would take about 3 to 3 ½ hours per day. She prescribed 60 mg prednisone for the swelling.

I could not take it all in. My thoughts were running a mile per minute. I called my children and told them about the tests results and what the doctor said. They were so concerned they told me that I should get a second opinion from another doctor.

I started taking prednisone, according to the doctor's instructions. Despite taking it, however, the swelling did not go down, instead it became worse. The swelling was so bad that at times, I had to take my hand and open my eyes. I could not see anything. There was so much excruciating aches and pains along with the swelling. Since I did not see where I was progressing, I started to question the doctor about his treatment of my sickness.

Overview Of Lupus

Lupus is a lifelong disorder of the immune system. With this disease, immune cells attack the body's own healthy tissues, leading to inflammation and tissue damage.

There are two kinds of lupus: Discoid lupus erythematosus (DLE) and Systemic lupus erythematosus (SLE). While DLE mainly affects skin that is exposed to sunlight and doesn't typically affect vital internal organs, SLE is more serious. It affects the skin and other vital organs.

Aside from the visible effects of systemic lupus, the disease may also inflame and/or damage the connective tissue in the joints, muscles, and skin, along with the membranes surrounding or within the lungs, heart, kidneys, and brain. SLE can also cause kidney disease (Lupus - Overview & Facts 2018).

According to Doctor Van Hook, I was diagnosed with Lupus SLE.

Chapter 3

Dealing With The Disease

The day after Dr. Van Hook referred me to the kidney specialist, I called Dr. Robert Lynn to get an appointment. I wanted to learn how the dialysis procedure works.

After consulting with him, he gave me a tour of the center and a date to do dialysis. I would have to go three days per week - Mondays, Wednesdays, and Fridays to do dialysis. However, I did not go. I was too scared of what I was dealing with.

The sickness started to progress. I was not able to return to work. My body became swollen all over. I could not wear any shoes. I had to wear oversized slippers and socks. After about one month of not doing the dialysis, I started fainting at home, several times.

I got even more scared of my sickness because of the frequent fainting spells. My children also got scared. They started crying and I had to ask them to stop. They were saying, "Look at what become of mom." They hired a home-help aide for me, through my insurance. Whenever I passed out at home my home-help aide would call the ambulance.

On one occasion when I was admitted to Montefiore Hospital, I realized that I had no choice but to do the dialysis treatment. I decided to regularly do dialysis as scheduled and recommended by the doctors.

For dialysis, they inserted a tube above my breast area and it stayed taped to my chest. It was very uncomfortable. It affected how I slept because it could pull apart. Once I was sitting, and my grandson told me that I was bleeding at my chest. I checked and saw that the tube for dialysis fell out. My daughter got a towel and wrapped it around me.

I slowly went to the emergency room at a close by hospital where I got treated. I called my doctor and he arranged for an ambulance to pick me up and take me to the Einstein hospital where he worked. I had to stay overnight until the dialysis tube got fixed. I was very uncomfortable. I could only lie in one painful position. Throughout all this trial I prayed within my mind and asked God to cover me, to give me strength, and to empower me to overcome the sickness.

My son, Lee, who lives in Florida was greatly grieved with my health situation. In 2009, he invited me to stay with him and his family for two weeks. I took him up on the offer. He and his wife came to New York and took me to Florida.

I got my medical records transferred them to the facility in Florida where I continued doing dialysis. I did the same schedule of three days per week. When I got back to New

York I felt so relaxed because I had been resting during my entire time in Florida.

It took a lot of patience to deal with this sickness and I had a lot of patience. My inner strength came from God. Sometimes I would burst out in tears. One time, while in New York, when I saw my coworker passing by on her way to work I burst in tears and asked God, "Why me? Why me?" In all the ups and downs of the disease, I always call on God. This gave me the strength I needed to carry on the fight.

No matter what you're going through never leave God out of your sickness or, whatever situation you may be dealing with…keep calling on His name.

Chapter 4

More Battles To Be Won

Even though I started doing dialysis on the recommended schedule and taking medication, the lupus disease continued to progress. It led to me having asthma, which is a wicked sickness. I was having shortness of breath. So, my struggle with severe sickness turned into two battles – one of the disease (enemy) more wicked than the other.

Little did I know that another enemy was on the way, due to asthma.

Because of the shortness of breath, I started having seizures. The third enemy had surfaced. The combination of all these sicknesses caused me to be in and out of the hospital. My grandchildren were staying with me and they kept panicking whenever they witnessed my asthma and seizures. I had to encourage them not to panic and call the ambulance. Most of the time when the ambulance came, my seizure was over.

Once, while having a seizure I had to call the ambulance to take me to the Emergency Room. I did not have time to tell anyone that I was going to the emergency room. I was in the hospital and no one knew where I was. I had an operation on my throat for thyroid problem, which made me unable to speak. I had a tracheal tube in my throat after the operation. I had to communicate with the doctor and nurse by writing on paper. I got some papers to sign. I also wrote the names and contact numbers for my friends and family members so that the nurse could call them to let them know where I was and what was going on with me. Later, when my children contacted me I also had to communicate with them through writing.

Another time, while at home making breakfast for my grandchildren, I was having a seizure and it lead to a minor stroke. When this happened, I found myself just making funny noises. While going through this, my daughter, Sophia, from New Jersey called and I could not talk. I could only say, "Amm, Amm."

My daughter called an ambulance and I was taken to the hospital. My grandchildren were at the house, so they had to go with me to the hospital. At the hospital, the nurse put a pill under my tongue. Immediately, I stopped saying, "Amm, Amm" when responding to anyone. Later, the doctors prescribe evetiracetam (keppra) 500 mg for the seizure and gave me an asthma pump to address the shortness of breath.

My daughter, Diane, visited me at the hospital and I could not recognize her. After I went to sleep and woke up my daughter was by my side. I called her name. Diane was so happy to see that I recognized her. She hugged me and told me she loved me. She started to cry.

I stayed in the hospital for two days, after which I was assigned a social worker. After returning home, the social worker came to my house to evaluate me. She wanted to see how I was walking, so she asked me to get up and walk. She was shocked to see me walking and talking. She said I was doing good and that I was so blessed. She told me that in all her work, I was the first patient she met who had a stroke and could still walk and talk. She concluded that I did not need therapy.

The social worker asked if I went to church. I told her, "Yes." She said that she could see why I recovered miraculously from the stroke and that I should just take care of myself.

During my dialysis treatment I was still going to church. I knew God kept me through one battle after the other with these multiple sicknesses. He has a purpose for me and I must fulfill His plan for my life. I thank God that He saved my life. I'm so grateful that I am still here.

I am encouraging others who are going through similar sicknesses not to give up. Please stay strong and fight the battle, no matter what it takes. You must go through the storm to come out strong. I am sending a message to both men and women not to give up with whatever sicknesses you are fighting. Fight through the storm. Never give up.

According to Isaiah 54:17, "No weapon that formed against thee shall prosper and every tongue that shall rise against thee in judgment thou shall condemn." At home, I prayed continuously to God for healing, health, and strength through the storm.

Satan did not like that I chose to clink to God throughout all my sickness. During my sickness, he decided to challenge my faith. One night I had a vision in which he came to me and showed me a wheel chair, a walking cane, and a walker. After showing me these, he showed me doctors, family, and friends. I knew in my spirit that he wanted me to accept what he was showing me. I got defiant in my spirit and refused. All I said to the Satan is, "I rebuke you with the blood of Jesus." I then continued to say, "The blood, the blood," repeated. I fought him all through my vision and overcame all his temptations.

I gathered strength by going to church to fellowship with other children of God. As I was going through all my pain, suffering, and sorrow, I was still attending the Ecclesia Ministries International church. It was headed by the Bishop Dr. Stephen Hutchinson. The Bishop, who is a great Pastor, gave numerous inspirational sermons that also helped me endured and regain my strength. It was like my prayers were being answered.

Chapter 5

Building My Inner Strength To Overcome

After being diagnosed with lupus and having kidney disease, I was taking about 13 different medications. It was a fearsome task to take all these medications. I always pray and sing before taking them. I needed God to give me the inner strength to deal with this task.

I had two special songs to sing before taking the medications. The first one is, "Through it all, I learn to trust in Jesus and learn to depend on His name."

The second one is, "Hear my cry and deliver me."

There are other songs I sang for encouragement. These are:

- "Let God and let God"
- "There is power in the name of Jesus"
- "I cannot walk without Him holding my hands"
- "He touched me and made me whole"
- "I must have the Savior with me for I dear not walk alone"

I not only sing and pray to get me through my sickness, but I also read selected scriptures, day and night, to strengthen me and encourage my heart. Some of my favorites were:

Scripture:

Psalm 30:12, "To the end that *my* glory may sing praise to thee, and not be silent. O LORD my God, I will give thanks unto thee forever."

What it means to me:

If God heals my body I will rejoice and give Him praise. I was calling forth my healing.

Scripture:

Psalm 3:8, "*Nor* for the pestilence *that* walketh in darkness; *nor* for the destruction *that* wasteth at noonday."

What it means to me:

No enemy can come around my house because my God is in control.

Scripture:

Psalm 23:6, "Surely goodness and mercy shall follow me all the days of my life: and I will dwell in the house of the LORD forever."

What it means to me:

I will continue to go into God's house and worship with His other children; to give Him praise and honor, as long as I live.

☆☆☆☆☆☆☆☆☆☆☆☆☆

Scripture:

Psalm 5:12, "For thou, LORD, wilt bless the righteous; with favour wilt thou compass him as *with* a shield."

What it means to me:

The shield meant that I have the covering of my God, despite the terrible sickness I was going through.

☆☆☆☆☆☆☆☆☆☆☆☆☆

Scripture:

Psalm 24:10, "Who is this King of glory? The LORD of hosts, he *is* the King of glory."

What it means to me:

The words of this verse mean to me, exactly what it says. I acknowledge that my God in the King of glory.

Scripture:

Psalm 37:17, "For the arms of the wicked shall be broken: but the LORD upholdeth the righteous."

What it means to me:

I know that my God upholds me and will save my life to do His work on this earth.

Scripture:

Psalm 51:19, "Then shalt thou be pleased with the sacrifices of righteousness, with burnt offering and whole burnt offering: then shall they offer bullocks upon thine altar."

What it means to me:

When my heart is right I know God will be pleased with me. My offering to Him is my praise and worship and reading of His Word.

☆☆☆☆☆☆☆☆☆☆☆☆

Scripture:

Psalm 62:8, "Trust in him at all times; ye people, pour out your heart before him: God *is* a refuge for us."

What it means to me:

I trust God always and I pour out my heart, my mind, and my soul to Him for I know that He can help me.

☆☆☆☆☆☆☆☆☆☆☆☆☆

Scripture:

Psalm 56:1, "Be merciful unto me, O God: for man would swallow me up; he fighting daily oppresseth me."

What it means to me:

I kept crying out to God to have mercy on me and not let this oppressing sickness overcome me.

☆☆☆☆☆☆☆☆☆☆☆☆☆

Scripture:

Psalm 46:11, "The LORD of hosts *is* with us; the God of Jacob *is* our refuge."

What it means to me:

I know that God is with me and that He is my refuge and strength, always.

☆☆☆☆☆☆☆☆☆☆☆

Scripture:

Psalm 139:14, 23, 24, "I will praise thee; for I am fearfully *and* wonderfully made: marvellous *are* thy works; and *that* my soul knoweth right well.

Search me, O God, and know my heart: try me, and know my thoughts:

And see if *there be any* wicked way in me, and lead me in the way everlasting."

What it means to me:

I acknowledge that God is my Creator and He knows how He created this body. I am crying out to Him to heal this body. I know His works are marvelous.

He knows my heart and I ask Him to search me and test my thoughts so that I can be led by Him.

Scripture:

Psalm 25:16-21, "Turn thee unto me, and have mercy upon me; for I *am* desolate and afflicted.

The troubles of my heart are enlarged: *O* bring thou me out of my distresses.

Look upon mine affliction and my pain; and forgive all my sins.

Consider mine enemies; for they are many; and they hate me with cruel hatred.

O keep my soul, and deliver me: let me not be ashamed; for I put my trust in thee.

Let integrity and uprightness preserve me; for I wait on thee."

What it means to me:

I call on God to show me His mercy in my distressing situation with sickness. I ask Him to look at my sickness. I am helpless, overwhelmed, in deep distress, and my sickness is going from bad to worse. I ask for healing; for God to feel my pain and forgive my sins.

☆☆☆☆☆☆☆☆☆☆☆☆

Scripture:

Psalm 43:5, "Why art thou cast down, O my soul? and why art thou disquieted within me? hope in God: for I shall yet praise him, *who is* the health of my countenance, and my God."

What it means to me:

These words encouraged me not to get into depression because my hope is in God. I speak to myself that, "God is my health despite what I am going through it. I know He will make me smile again, for He is my God."

☆☆☆☆☆☆☆☆☆☆☆☆

Scripture:

Isaiah 54:17, "No weapon that is formed against thee shall prosper; and every tongue *that* shall rise against thee in judgment thou shalt condemn. This *is* the heritage of the servants of the LORD, and their righteousness *is* of me, saith the LORD."

What it means to me:

I know that this sickness I am going through will not overcome me. I claim this as a child of God.

Scripture:

Psalm 18:19-20, "He brought me forth also into a large place; he delivered me, because he delighted in me.

The LORD rewarded me according to my righteousness; according to the cleanness of my hands hath he recompensed me."

What it means to me:

In all my struggle with sickness I continually call on God to deliver me. His deliverance from my sickness came when He allowed a man to donate his kidney which was a match for me. This man's kidney is my reward from God for holding on to Him during such brutal battles with multiple sicknesses. God has done this for me, because I did right by Him during my period of trials and tribulations – I did not give up on Him, but faced all my situations, while holding onto Him.

Chapter 6

The Great Victory

In June 2013, I applied for donor kidney at two hospitals while going through dialysis. A Sunday in November of the same year, while I was on the dialysis machine, I got a call from Mt. Sinai Hospital that a live donor was giving a kidney which matched mine. I must say, I was as calm as a dove when I heard the news.

A nurse said to me, "You should be rejoicing." I just quietly thanked God. I did not want to tell too many people about this. On previous occasions, when I would get a call that they got a kidney for me I would quickly tell my family. In the end, the promise of kidney would get cancelled and I would be very disappointed about not getting it.

After I was done with the dialysis, I simply called my daughter to take me home. At home, I got a shower and then asked her to take me downtown to a hospital to see a nurse who wanted to talk to me. I did not share with her that I was going for a new kidney.

Discovering The Misdiagnosis

I went to the Mount Sinai hospital in Manhattan, New York, where the doctors began to conduct a series of blood tests to determine my blood type and to see if my blood type was compatible with the kidney that I was receiving from a donor. As a result, the doctors determined that it was a perfect match.

Next, the doctors checked my body in the kidney area to examine where they were going to lay the kidney. They began to clean the kidney thoroughly and told me to prepare myself for the kidney transplant operation. It was at the hospital that my daughter, Nashera, found out I was getting a kidney. She got curious about all the activities that were going on with me. She asked the nurse what was going on and the nurse told her that I got a kidney from a donor. My daughter cried with joy.

While waiting on the specific blood test, one of the doctors reviewing the results came in the room in a hurry. He was a Caucasian man and he became red in the face with anger. He said, "Miss Robertson, who diagnosed you with lupus?" I told him doctor Van Hook. He asked for the doctor's number and I gave it to him. He called doctor Van Hook and asked her why she diagnosed me with lupus when I did not have lupus. This doctor was so upset that he did not come back to me.

Another doctor came in and told me he just came out of a meeting about me. He told me I was diagnosed with the wrong sickness and asked if I was taking medication. I told him, "Yes." He told me not to take it anymore. I thought,

"Oh my God! I am taking the wrong medication in my body."

Furthermore, I realized that the medications (mycophemol, 500 mg) that I was taking for lupus had greatly contributed to the problems and complications I was experiencing initially. The side effects were excruciating pain, swellings in the face, feet and hands, dizziness, drowsiness, fainting, loss of appetite, among others. Those medications did not make me feel well and I could ever relax. I felt as if I was living in a torture chamber. I felt like a walking zombie.

I tried not to keep reflecting on the compounded problems I had due to wrong diagnosis and wrong medication. I had to focus on relaxing to receive the new kidney. A team of doctors conducted the kidney transplant. The operation was a success.

After I went home, I threw out all the medications I was taking for lupus. Although I was displeased with the doctor who diagnosed me with lupus and had me taking medication for it, the greater joy of having a new kidney and a new lease on life overshadowed that.

I told my daughter, Nasheria, that I found out I did not have lupus. I related the full story to her. She called the doctor who had mis-diagnosed me with lupus. However, no one answered the phone. She called on numerous occasion to no avail.

Recovery With The New Kidney

My health improved drastically with the new kidney. There was no more swelling in my body. It worked beautifully. There was no reaction to it. My body adjusted perfectly. I did not have to do another dialysis during the normal adjustment period.

In some of my previous dialysis sessions, some people would come during their adjustment periods to do dialysis, after kidney transplant.

I felt elated, more like a new person. I thank God for giving me the chance to live a healthy life once again. I had never given up on Him during my terrible ordeal with what was supposed to be lupus disease but turned out to be purely kidney disease.

I am rejoicing and thanking God every day for allowing me to get this kidney. It was from a live male donor about 20 years younger than me. I thank God for him.

Bibliography

Lupus - Overview & Facts. *WebMD*,
    17 September 2018,
        https://www.webmd.com/lupus/g
        uide/lupus-overview-facts

The Holy Bible. King James Version.
    Holman Bible Publishers, 1979.

9 781724 193759